# The D●T METHOD

## an interactive tool to teach kids about cancer

# The D●T METHOD
## an interactive tool to teach kids about cancer

Kelsey Mora, CCLS, LCPC

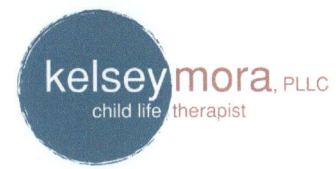

Kelsey Mora, PLLC
Northfield, Illinois

www.childlifetherapist.com | @the.dot_method

ISBN-13: 979-8-9890005-0-0

Edited by Allison Kessel Clark

Printed in the United States of America

The content in this book is for informational purposes only. It is not intended to be a substitute for professional medical advice and should not be relied upon as health or personal advice.

Always seek the guidance of your doctor or other qualified health professional with any questions you may have regarding your health or a medical condition. Never disregard the advice of a medical professional or delay seeking it because of something you read here.

Dedicated with love to my dear friends, the Welker family, and to all the families who I have had the honor and privilege to walk alongside and support throughout their cancer experience.

# PRAISE FOR *THE DOT METHOD*

"Kelsey Mora has done something that has been missing in the medical field for a long, long time—creating a comprehensive guidebook to navigating cancer."
Gina Moffa, LCSW

"When a patient receives a cancer diagnosis, they are thrown into having to learn so many things with almost no aid outside a short office visit. This tool takes the unmet need of how to talk about cancer with your children off the list."
Sanjay Juneja, MD

"As a mom with incurable cancer, I will use *The Dot Method* to help guide conversations with my children and provide them with a visual of the effects of my daily treatment."
Michelle Hughes, mother

"The idea of using this creative method, straight forward tool, and queries to envision what is unimaginable or unexplainable crafts clarity, understanding, and plain language that is so needed when cancer enters the conversation and a life. This method is an every-body gift."
Barri Leiner Grant, grief coach

"Dealing with cancer is hard enough. Talking about it with your kids shouldn't be. That's why every parent NEEDS *The Dot Method.*"
Em Jamieson, RN, BSN, CHPN, OCN

"This approach helped me explain treatment to my toddler who did not know what cancer was. Kelsey's method helped her see things in an age-appropriate way, and made an impossible time a little more digestible for her."
Danielle Moss, mother and childhood cancer advocate

# CONTENTS

# A NOTE TO THE USER

Dear parent, caregiver, or trusted adult,

This is an opportunity to teach your child coping skills that are transferable to everyday life. Throughout my work with children and adolescents impacted by cancer and other life-altering events, I have developed three consistent and necessary messages that I like to share with parents and caregivers:

➤ **Honesty really is the best policy:** Children pick up on cues in their environment. They look to their trusted adults to try to make sense of things they are observing and experiencing. Instead of avoiding a topic, you can build trust by creating a space and an environment where all topics, including cancer, are acceptable and safe to discuss. Open communication also helps to give kids a truthful narrative about the situation rather than leaving them to make sense of things on their own.

➤ **When in doubt, keep things "normal":** Children benefit from routine, structure, and predictability. These things help to give children a sense of control and stability when life feels out of control and unpredictable. Prepare children for anticipated changes and expectations, and aim to keep some aspects of their childhood as normal as possible. Parents who are facing cancer themselves also benefit from continuing to parent their child through typical growth and development, as it provides the parent a much-needed sense of normalcy.

➤ **Expressing feelings is healthy:** By naming and sharing your own feelings, you have the potential to teach your child about safe and effective expression of all emotions, even the uncomfortable ones. All feelings are okay; some behaviors are not. This is an opportunity to teach your child transferrable coping skills.

Although I wish that you did not need this book, my hope is that it can provide you with a tool to explain and teach children about cancer in a non-threatening, interactive, and playful way that is led and created from your own unique and personal experience.

Best wishes,
Kelsey Mora

# HOW TO USE THIS WORKBOOK

**1. Preview the Workbook**

Familiarize yourself with the book layout and the method before presenting the book to a child. A summary of the method is shown on pages 20-21. Preview the Glossary. Think about the questions presented throughout, and consider how the child in your care might respond. Be prepared for a variety of answers. No two children will have the same exact questions nor responses, as no two scenarios are exactly the same. You know your child best.

**2. Know Your Audience**

This workbook was designed to be used with all ages and cancer relationships. Strive to look at the book together; working through the book with a trusted adult encourages discussion, deepens understanding, and strengthens expression. Always use words that match the child's age and experience, and modify as appropriate.

For maximum success when presenting *The Dot Method*, use these ideas as guides:

**Ages 0-4:** While the ideas and vocabulary may be too advanced for this age group, understanding *The Dot Method* in its simplest form is still possible. Consider using one of the blank outlines at the back of the book to present the method simply and visually.

**Ages 5-6:** Children at this age may rely on you for reading. They may ask a lot of questions. Simplify language as needed, with a focus specifically on healthy cells, unhealthy/cancer cells, and medicine/treatment.

**Ages 7-10:** Children at this age may be able to read and understand concepts more independently. Your job is to explain any confusing concepts, encourage discussion, and provide support.

**Ages 11 and above:** While this workbook is geared for younger children, older children will still benefit. An older child can complete the workbook with little or no reading assistance, but interactive use with an adult is optimal. Act as a guide or support and use open-ended questions to prompt and encourage the sharing of feelings.

**3. Understand Your Comfort Level**

People have different comfort levels when it comes to the word *cancer*. Although using the term can be helpful to ensure children understand how cancer is different from other illnesses, it can feel scary and uncomfortable for some. This book is meant as a guide, and parents or caregivers should feel comfortable throughout the workbook exchanging the word *cancer* for *unhealthy* or *broken cells*, if preferred.

## 4. Choose Your Preferred Media or Materials

*The Dot Method* can be completed using crayons, colored pencils, or markers, but it can also be done using different colored pom-poms or small tangible circle items if you have a tactile learner. One advantage to completing the book using physical items is that you or the child can use the book over and over again to review, learn more, and teach others along the way. Note that additional blank outlines are at the back of the workbook for your convenience.

## 5. Present the Workbook

Use the questions shown on each page as a guide to interact with the child through the learning process. Always encourage discussion. Allow the child to decide whether or not to share his or her work and learning. Know that sometimes you might not have an answer for a question. This is ok and normal. Sometimes the best response is simply saying, "That is a great question. I don't know the answer, but when I do, I'll discuss it with you" or "Let's find out together."

# GLOSSARY

Use this section as a guide to further explain terms as needed.

**cancer** - an illness that occurs when someone's body develops unhealthy cells that grow, multiply, or even take up space. Every cancer has a different name that often describes the location of the cancer cells in the body. Because cancer is not caused by germs, you can't catch it like a cold.

**cells** - one of the smallest units that makes up an organism. Cells are so tiny that they can be seen only through a microscope, but they make up the entire body including skin, blood, and organs.

**chemotherapy or chemo** - a strong medicine that attacks cancer cells and helps to get rid of them. Chemo can be taken by mouth or through a tube called an IV or a port. Chemo is so strong that it can cause side effects, like making a person feel unhealthy or tired, or changing how the person looks.

**coping skills** - actions and strategies a person uses to help deal with difficult situations or uncomfortable feelings in order to feel calmer.

**hospital** - the place where medical procedures and treatment often take place. Sometimes people spend the night in a hospital, and sometimes people visit a clinic for just a few hours.

**immunocompromised** - when the immune system becomes weakened from treatment and has a harder time fighting off germs that can cause contagious diseases or infections, we might use this term to describe that person.

**immunotherapy** - a type of treatment that can be taken by mouth or through a tube that helps a person's immune system attack the cancer cells. It can stop or slow the growth of the cancer so that the immune system becomes better at getting rid of the cancer cells.

**IV** - "IV" stands for *intravenous,* which literally means "inside the vein." An IV is a small tube or straw placed in a person's vein, where the blood lives. This tube is used to give medicines and fluids to a patient. It is placed each time the person needs medicine, and it remains in place only in the hospital or medical office.

**medicine** - a broad term for substances like a liquid, pill, or tablet used to treat a medical problem to help a person get better. Some examples include chemotherapy and pain relievers.

**port** - a device placed under the skin during surgery that can then be used as a spot to insert medicine and draw blood through a tube into the body. It is usually on the person's chest and stays until the person is done needing medicine.

**radiation** - a type of treatment. Radition enters the body through a beam of energy, an injection, or ingestion. Radiation targets a specific part of the body and makes the cancer smaller. Radiation can make a person feel unhealthy, tired, or sore.

**side effects** - symptoms that can happen to a person as a result of treatment and medicine. A person might feel tired, weak, or nauseous. Side effects are different for everyone.

**surgery** - when doctors work on a problem inside or on someone's body. The doctor first gives medicine called *anesthesia* to help the person sleep and not feel pain. Surgery can be to remove, reduce, or test the cancer or tumor, as well as to prepare a person for treatment.

**symptoms** - signs that the body gives to signal that something is not right. Some symptoms are serious; some are not.

**treatment** - a broad term that includes the different types of care given to a cancer patient. This can include surgery, chemotherapy, radiation, and immunotherapy.

**tumor or mass** - when cancer cells take up space in the body, they can get stuck together and create something called a *tumor* or *mass*. This does not always happen, and not every tumor is made up of cancer cells.

# THE DOT METHOD

Illnesses come in many types. Some can be caused by germs, bacteria, or viruses.

Many illnesses can be treated at home. Other illnesses require the use of special medicines, doctors, or nurses.

**What illnesses do you already know about? Draw or write about them here.**

Everyone's body is made up of millions of tiny healthy cells doing different jobs. You can't see cells, but they are in the skin, the blood, and the organs.

**Choose a color. Use this color to show healthy cells. Make dots all over the body in that color.**

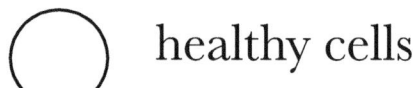 healthy cells

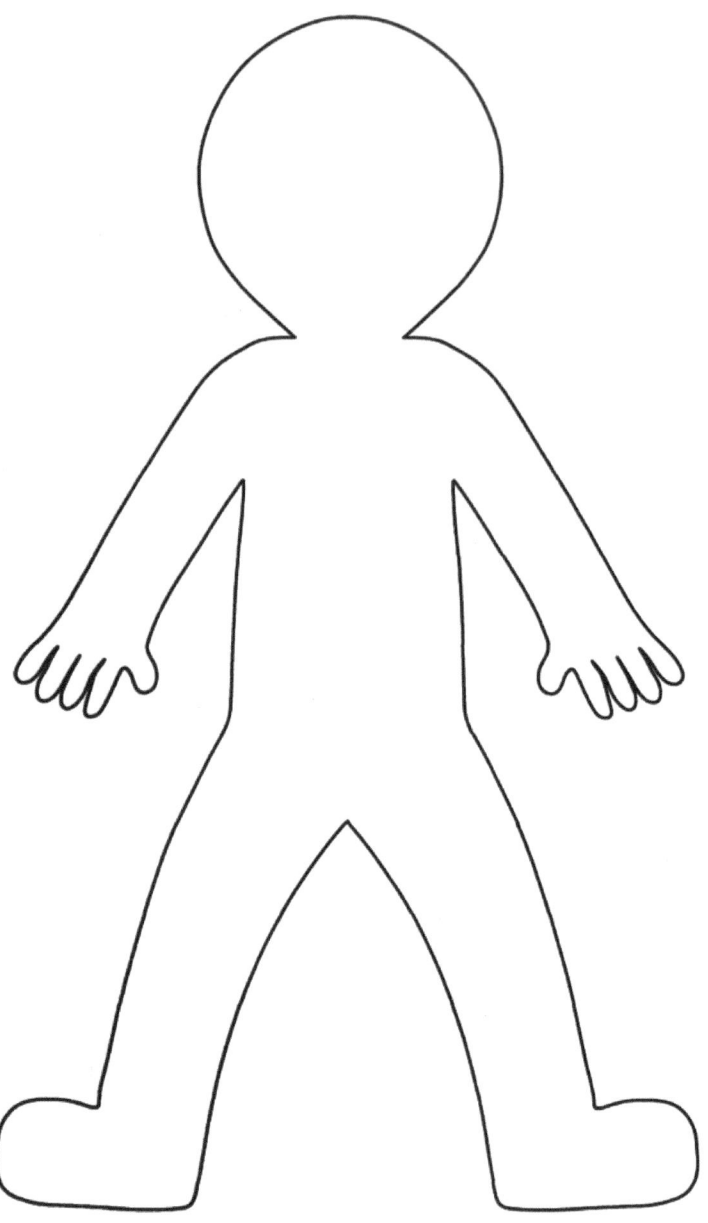

Symptoms are signs that there might be a problem with someone's health. Some symptoms are serious. Some are not. A doctor or hospital can run tests that help identify if there is a problem.

The tests might show extra cells that aren't supposed to be in the body. These extra cells might be unhealthy or broken.

**What medical tests have you heard of? Draw them or write them on the line.**

Here are some ideas to help you get started:

CT scan                              ultrasound

MRI                                  blood work

_____

Have you heard the word *cancer* before? Cancer can happen when cells do not do their job correctly. And when cells don't do their job, they can cause problems for the whole body.

Do you know someone who has or had cancer? **Write that person's name.**

_____

**Use the body outline to create that person.**

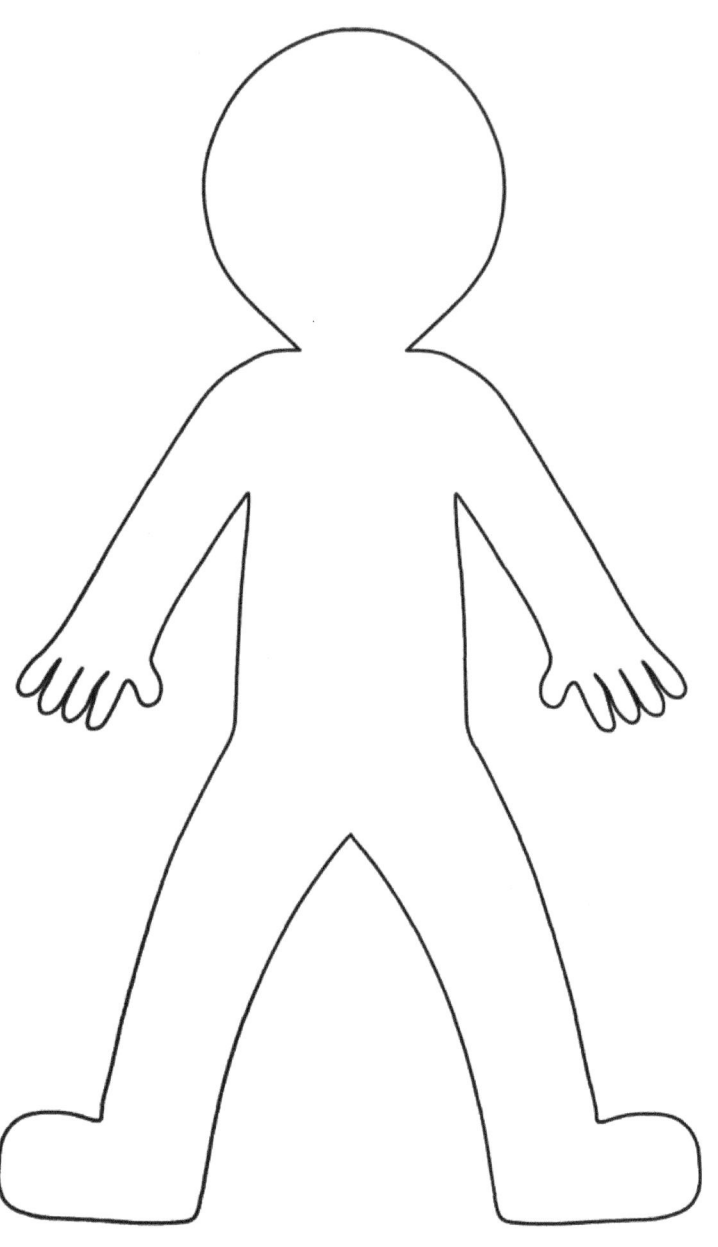

It's important to know…

- You can't see cancer cells with your eyes.
- You can't catch cancer from someone.
- No one caused the cells to get unhealthy or broken.
- Sometimes cancer just happens.
- Everyone's cancer experience is different.

**What questions do you have? Write them below.**

Remember what color you used to show healthy cells. Now choose a different color to represent cancer cells.

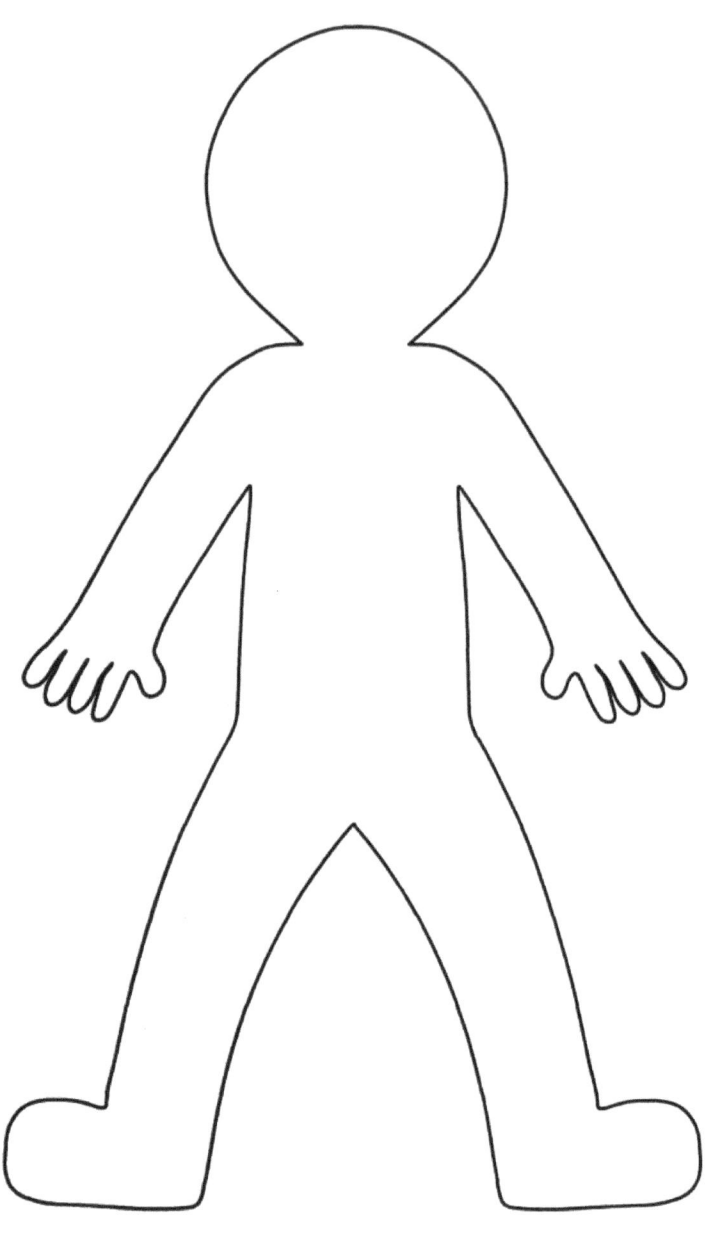

○ cancer cells

When cancer cells stick together in one area, we call it a *tumor* or a *mass*.

Using the color above, show cancer cells by making dots inside the body.

**Draw extra cancer cells in one spot if there is a specific part of the body where the person has cancer.**

There are many different types of cancer. Each type of cancer requires a different type of treatment or medicine.

Treatment might be surgery. Or it might be medicine. Or it might be a combination of both.

Treatment happens in a hospital or medical facility. Doctors, nurses, and surgeons are the ones who give treatment.

**Draw a picture of a hospital or place where somebody goes to receive treatment.**

Surgery is one type of cancer treatment.

Surgery can be done to test cells. Or surgery might be done to remove a cancer mass or make it smaller.

Radiation is another type of treatment. Radiation can enter the body through a beam of energy. Or it can enter the body like a medicine through a vein or the mouth.

Did your person have surgery or radiation? **Circle your answer.**

yes                              no

Medicine is another type of cancer treatment.

Two common medicines are *chemotherapy* and *immunotherapy*. A person might have one or both.

These treatments can enter the body through
a tube called a *port*,
a tube called an *IV*, or
the person's mouth as a pill or a liquid.

Sometimes a person might need a combination of different types of treatments.

Does the person you know need one or more? **Circle your answer.**

surgery        radiation        medicine        other

Let's learn about how treatment works.

First, draw healthy cell dots and cancer cell dots. Use the same colors you used before. Choose a new color for treatment.

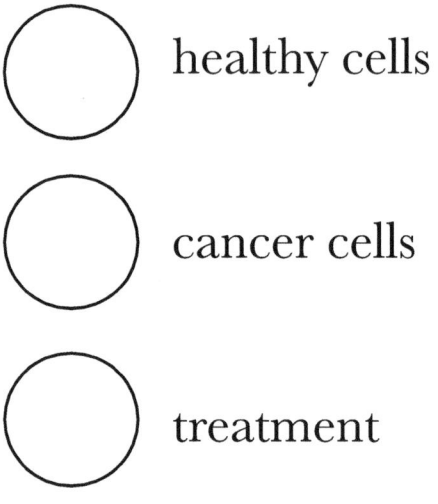 healthy cells

cancer cells

treatment

Treatment can be used to get rid of or fix as many cancer cells as possible.

**Using your treatment color, draw an X through the cancer cells.**

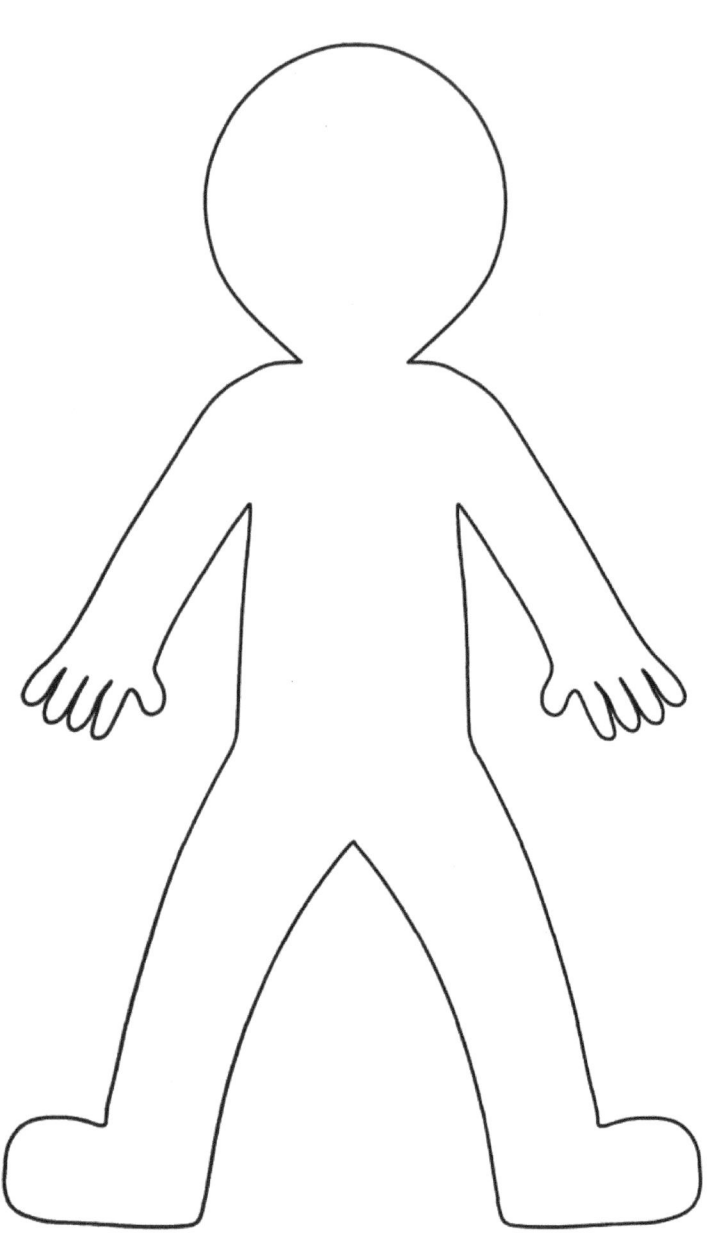

Sometimes the treatment gets rid of all the cancer cells. Sometimes it gets rid of just some of the cancer cells. And sometimes it keeps cells from growing or multiplying.

Treatment medicine is strong. It's so strong that it sometimes even damages healthy cells.

**Go back and draw an X through some of the healthy cells using your treatment color.**

The healthy cells can recover. But when healthy cells get damaged, a person may experience side effects. These are some common side effects that a person might have:

- feeling tired, sore, or nauseous,
- losing hair,
- being *immunocompromised*, which means "more susceptible to germs"

This is normal, and it means the medicine is working hard.

Does the person you know have side effects? **Write or draw those things below.**

It's normal for the medicine to make a person feel unhealthy or tired some days. It's also normal for a person to feel well and healthy some days.

Some activities are good for when a person is having a good day. Other activities are good for when a person is not feeling well. **Draw or write about those activities here. What ideas do you have for each type of day?**

GOOD DAY | DIFFICULT DAY

Each person's cancer experience is unique.

Sometimes the cancer goes away.

Sometimes the cancer won't go away, and the person needs treatment throughout life.

No one experiences cancer alone. Doctors, nurses, scientists, family, and friends work together as a team. They help and support the entire family. Sometimes they help by giving treatment. Sometimes they help by looking for new medicines. Sometimes they help by enjoying time together.

Everyone has the same goal: to get rid of the cancer. When that's not possible, the goal is to keep the cancer cells small, treat side effects, and help the person continue to enjoy life as long as possible.

**Write your questions about treatment or goals. These are different for everyone.**

It's normal to have different feelings about cancer. What feelings do you have?

**Draw different faces in the circles below. Write the name of the feeling next to the face.**

◯ _____

◯ _____

◯ _____

◯ _____

It's normal to have uncomfortable or hard feelings. Some people feel better when they talk to or spend time with others.

Who are some people that make you feel better just by talking or being with them? **Write their names or draw their pictures below.**

We all want to understand cancer better and to know how to treat it. Learning about cancer and talking about it are important first steps.

Cancer causes people to have questions. This is normal. The person who has cancer has questions. And the people around that person have questions too.

Not all questions have simple answers.

Look back at the questions you had on page 5. Which ones were answered? What questions do you still have? **Write them below and ask an adult.**

Even when someone you love has cancer, you still have reasons to experience joy, to be happy, and to have fun with the people you love.

Sometimes we do things specifically to help ourselves feel calmer. We call those actions *coping skills*.

**Draw or write about something you do that makes you feel calmer or happier.**

Cancer can be scary and unpredictable. But there are many ways you can help yourself.

Talk to someone.

Ask questions.

Learn more from people you trust.

Use coping skills.

Keep doing things that are important to you.

Remember how treatment works using The Dot Method.

**Put a checkmark next to the ways that are your favorite.**

To review how treatment works, remember The Dot Method. Just follow these steps:

**1. First, draw a body outline.**

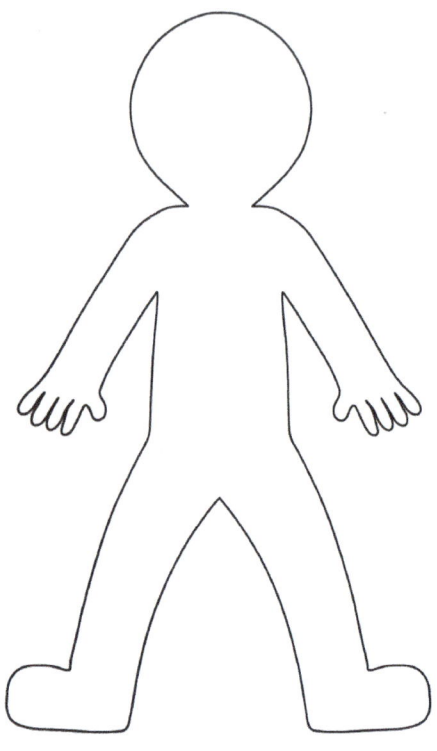

**2. Next, draw healthy cell dots.**

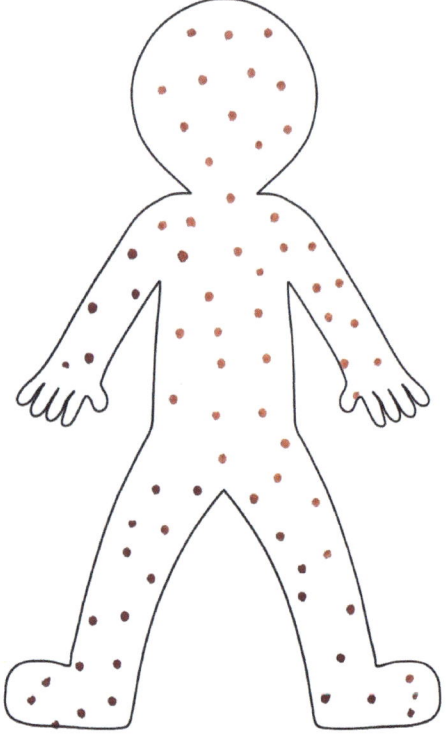

20

## 3. Then draw cancer cell dots.

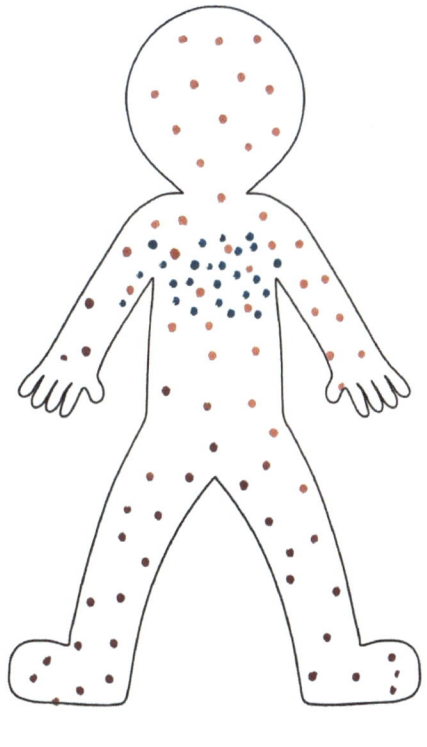

## 4. Finally, cross out many cancer cell dots and some healthy cell dots to show how treatment works.

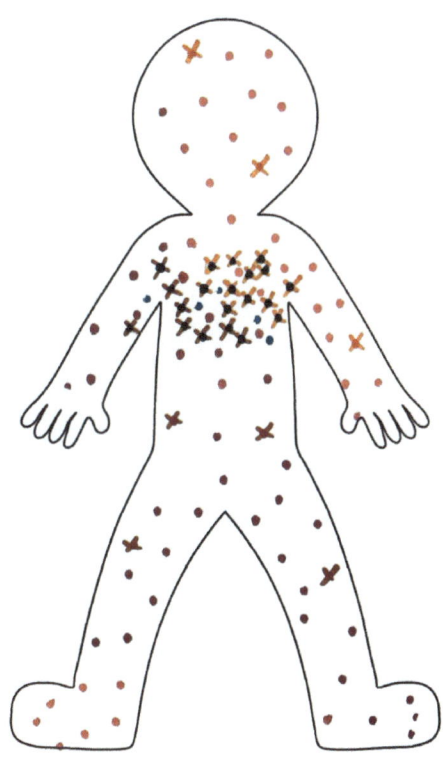

And remember, you are not alone in this journey.

# EXTRA OUTLINES

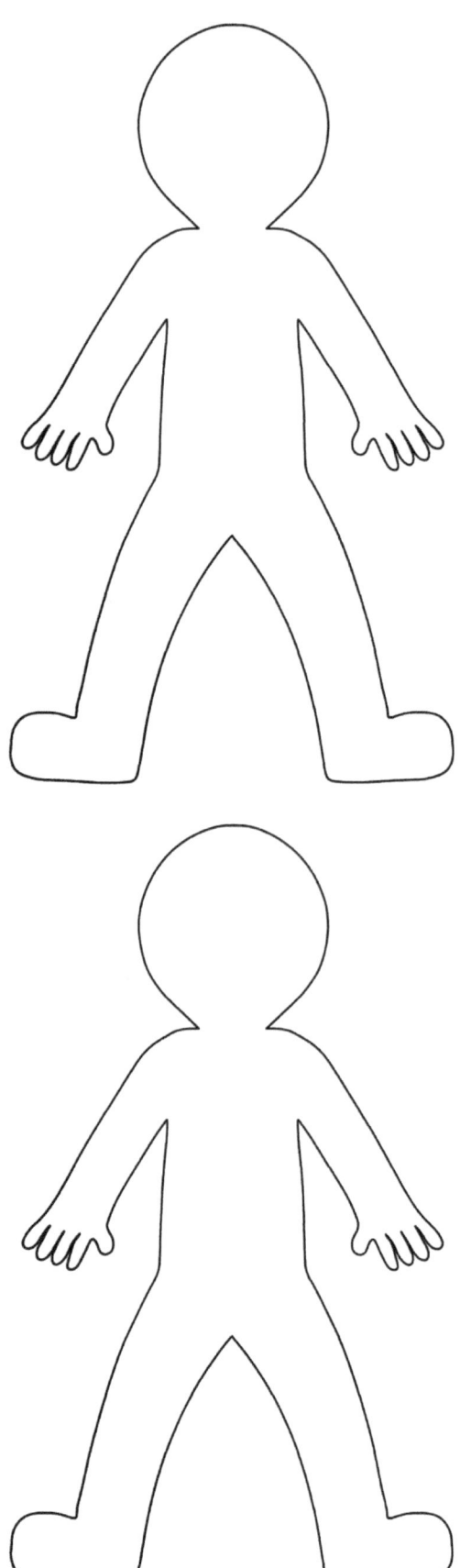
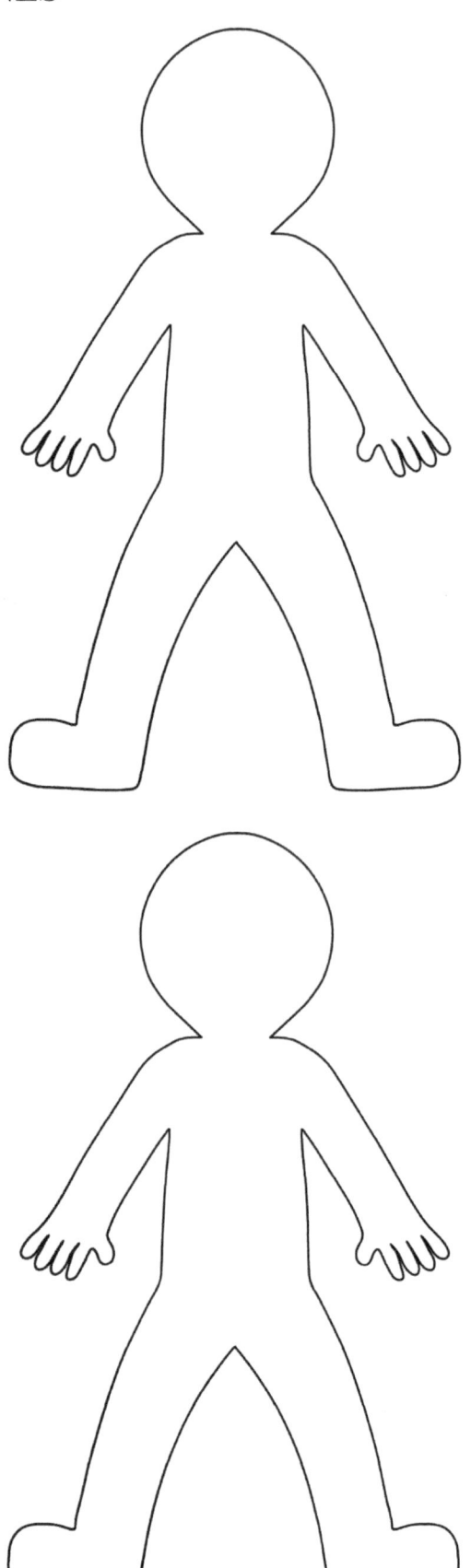

# ABOUT THE AUTHOR

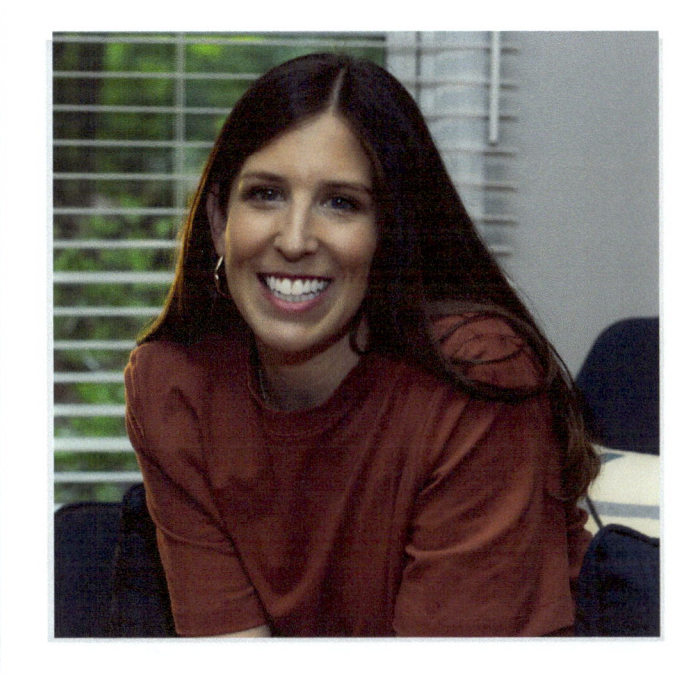

Kelsey Mora is a dual-certified child life specialist and licensed clinical professional counselor practicing in the Chicagoland area. Ms. Mora is specifically trained not only to support children and adolescents individually, but also to guide caregivers on how to deliver difficult news to the children in their care.

Ms. Mora has developed **The Method Workbooks** series for delivering specific types of difficult information to children. The first of these methods is *The Dot Method*, which is an intervention designed to educate children about cancer using honest, age-appropriate language and a play-based approach. This book is intended to be used by children and a trusted adult together. The tool can be used in various settings, from healthcare environments to therapy to home.

Ms. Mora is available for consultations and presentations on illness, grief, and other life stressors. She can be reached at kelsey@childlifetherapist.com or through her Instagram account: @childlifetherapist .

Interested in sharing your child's work and seeing how others cope and learn using *The Dot Method?* Take a photo of your child's drawing, upload it to social media, and tag it with @themethodworkbooks and #thedotmethod.